Well RN

The healthy lifestyle guide for nurses

By Caryn L. Haywood, MS, RDN

Haywood Health

Well RN: The healthy lifestyle guide for nurses
First edition paperback
ISBN: 978-0-578-63242-1

Published in the United States of America by:

Haywood Health
16751 Sheridan Street #159
Fort Lauderdale, FL 33331

To order a copy of this book, please email:
caryn@carynhaywood.com

Disclaimer: The content in this book is for educational and information purposes. It is not a substitute or replacement for professional medical advice. Consult your physician before starting any new diet or exercise program.

For Nadine

Foreward

Welcome to Well RN! My name is Caryn L. Haywood, Registered Dietitian Nutritionist. Most of my career has been in clinical nutrition.
Before earning my master's degree in dietetics and nutrition, I was a health educator for a public school in grades 9-12. While teaching, I discovered that I had a particular fondness of teaching the unit on nutrition. My creativity seemed to spike when I had to plan my nutrition lessons. I wanted to engage the teens to see how proper nutrition is just as important as saying no to drugs.
I left the classroom to pursue a career as a registered dietitian because I saw how childhood obesity and lifestyle-related diseases were quickly becoming a public health problem in our country, and I wanted to be a part of the solution. I was intrigued by the diversity of opportunities in the career of dietetics and nutrition.
While in graduate school, I started volunteering with a local non-profit organization teaching community nutrition classes to all ages. It gave me so much joy to help others by sharing my knowledge of proper nutrition.

I earned a certificate of training in adult weight management from the Commission of Dietetic Registration to continue strengthening my nutrition counseling skills.

One-on-one counseling seemed to be a challenge to manage when you are trying to serve nurses that work twelve-hour shifts. The idea for this book came about when I realized I could connect with so many more busy professionals by creating a healthy lifestyle guide tailored to their career. Take what you have learned and apply it to your life. I would love to hear your success stories. Please share with the hashtag, #WellRN.

I thank you for the opportunity to help improve your lifestyle and help you become the best version of you.

TABLE OF CONTENTS

Part 1

Introduction

The Well RN guide is for all nurses, inspired by the nurses that I have had the pleasure to work with during my career as a registered dietitian. When I started working in the hospital, I quickly formed friendly relationships with the nurses on the unit, and they would often confide in me their struggles to maintain a healthy lifestyle, as well as personal difficulties with nutrition courses in school.

It became clear to me that the nursing profession is nurturing, and for some nurses, that comes at an expense at the nurse's health.
I know how critical nurses are to the overall care of a patient; however, personal care is the foundation of thriving in any career or life in general.

The goal of the Well RN guide is to provide nurses with practical strategies to balance personal health and a successful nursing career. With so many responsibilities at home and work, it can be challenging to see how self-care fits in, especially daily. Learning strategies with the RN's daily duties in mind will transform how you view your current work-life balance.

This book is a resource that you can refer back to for information and inspiration. Please email caryn@carynhaywood.com with feedback. I appreciate your input for future editions.

The Nursing Profession

As a nurse, you care for those who cannot care for themselves. You take on the role of a teacher, counselor, and often, family for the ill. You make an invaluable contribution to your community. However, some days you wake up and don't like how you feel or what you see in the mirror...or on the scale...or in your blood work results. You wonder how you got here and reminisce about the days when you felt more control over lifestyle choices probably before you became a nurse. Then the 12-hour shifts started. Three days on, four days off, right? Sure, for a while. Then life happened, and it became harder to make ends meet with just one job, or you decided to go back to school. You picked up extra shifts or enrolled in school to advance your career. Maybe you started a family. You thought the extra shifts were going to bring in more money, and you weren't expecting those 20 extra pounds. Those late-night study sessions are the perfect opportunity to indulge in comfort food, and snacks. Also, who keeps leaving sweets in the break room?!

How did that extra weight get there? You feel like you are either too tired or too busy at work to eat. Plus, you are always on your feet. No sedentary work here! Let's not get started on your responsibilities at home. Still, those extra pounds

are there, and it's starting to show in your blood pressure and lab work.
As a nurse, you probably feel that added layer of guilt on top of the displeasure with your unhealthy eating and lifestyle habits. You feel uncomfortable advising patients to adopt healthier habits when you know you are not actively taking your advice. You feel like a hypocrite.
You have tried different diet programs, like shakes, restrictive diets, maybe even a "medically supervised" weight loss program. They all worked until you stopped the program, and the weight came right back.

What about your family? Does more than one member of your household struggle with maintaining a healthy weight or a balanced diet? Are you struggling with what kinds of meals to prepare for your family?

Some of these challenges are a lack of nutrition education, lifestyle choices, or a combination of both. You have more control over your health than you might think. In this book, we will discuss being proactive with your diet and lifestyle choices.

For example, cultural preferences and traditions play a large part in meal choices and perceived resistance to change. Diets high starches like rice and beans, legumes can be modified to be more balanced while still preserving tradition.

Even the busiest of moms can find time to fit some time to exercise a few times a week. Note that I did not put a duration or assign an activity to that statement. You will be required to reflect on your current daily habits and reduce or eliminate activities that you may not realize are major time wasters. Have you ever spent thirty minutes or more on Facebook or Instagram while lying in bed or sitting on the couch? Guess what? You could have put on some comfortable clothes and done a twenty-minute workout at home or gone for a walk.

Now is the time to wake up every morning and make a conscious decision to become the person you want to be. Get in the driver's seat of your health. You make hundreds, if not thousands of choices daily. Creating healthy habits makes some of those decisions almost automatic.

Think about your last great accomplishment. Was it completing nursing school and passing the NCLEX? Think about the energy that you put into reaching this goal. Remember the discipline that is required. Remember all the setbacks from which you recovered. Remember all the times you had to say no to things you much rather have been doing, but your desire to accomplish this goal was much higher than the temporary pleasure of a night out with friends or a weekend vacation. As the young people say these days, keep that same energy in wanting to be the best RN that you can be. That starts with proper self-care.

Before we get into what you want to change, let's recognize that you are a whole and complete person, just as you are. You are valuable just the way you are. Like I said before, we are all a work in progress. No one said it would be easy, but with time and self-discipline, the change will come.

You are reading this for a reason. You have one or more things in mind that you want to change regarding your health and current lifestyle. You must also know the reason why, and it must come from a personal desire, not someone else.
From speaking with nurses, I have found career-related challenges the come up frequently are:

1. Hydration
2. Lack of energy or time for exercise
3. Proper meal planning

What is holding you back?

This is probably not the first time you have tried to fix these areas of concern in your life. Think about previous attempts to change and why you think you did not succeed. If this is your first real attempt to take action, what has held you back from starting before this moment?

Key Points

- Nurses are amazing!
- Nursing is a physically and mentally challenging profession
- Self-care becomes a priority when you create lasting lifestyle habits

Part 2

Macronutrients

Carbohydrates

Let's face this so-called monster, head-on. How many nutrition courses did you take in nursing school? Maybe one? It's perfectly acceptable for you to pick up your phone and call the dietitian's office for diet education when a patient asks more than two questions about their diabetic menu. I get it; you need to give insulin and move on to the dressing change in the next room before the CNA has to go on break!

Carbohydrates are our body's preferred source of energy. They provide four calories per gram. All foods contain carbohydrates, but some have significantly more than others that can impact glycemic control in the body. Those are grains, legumes, fruits, milk, yogurt, and some vegetables. When reading nutrition labels, we need to look at total carbohydrate content, total fiber, as well as sugar content. The sugar content can be misleading, depending on the product. Sugar content from a bottle of 100% juice will be a lot different from a package of whole wheat bread. New nutrition facts labels include "added sugars," which is vital to know. You may be surprised to see added sugars in foods that you may not even consider to be sweet or needing sugar. Reading the ingredient list is just as important.

What is fiber?
Fiber is a form of carbohydrate that consists of two categories: Soluble and insoluble. Soluble fiber absorbs water like a sponge and turns into a gel, causing fullness. If you aren't drinking enough fluids, you may experience some very uncomfortable gastrointestinal symptoms. Insoluble fiber passes through the intestines undigested and adds bulk to the stool.

Why do I need fiber?
Your immune system is heavily concentrated in your intestines, and fiber consumption helps to protect the delicate balance of intestinal microbes. Fermentation of fiber in the intestines produces butyrate, the primary energy source for the large intestine. Butyrate helps to maintain the integrity of the intestinal lining. Compromised intestinal mucosa puts you more at risk for disease. Fiber can also help lower cholesterol and regulate blood sugar. Are you trying to lose weight? A diet rich in soluble fiber promotes the feeling of fullness and can help prevent overeating. Lastly, insoluble fiber helps to move waste through your colon and out of your body.

"I was diagnosed with inflammatory bowel disease and was told to eat a low fiber diet."

If you have IBD (Crohn's or Colitis) or irritable bowel syndrome (IBS), soft, cooked vegetables without seeds are more your speed.

What foods have fiber, and how much do I need? Soluble fiber exists in oat bran, apples, citrus fruit, nuts, seeds, beans, lentils, barley, and psyllium. Insoluble fiber exists in whole grains, vegetables, and wheat bran. Dietary fiber naturally occurring in minimally processed foods is always the best to get the recommended 25-35g fiber daily. Fresh or lightly cooked fruits and vegetables and whole grains should be a staple in your diet.

What about fiber supplements?
Conventional fiber dietary supplements come in the form of chicory root, inulin, psyllium. Fiber is added to many food products like multivitamins, snack foods, protein powders, and various other nutrition supplements. Fiber-fortified food products may be the culprit of those aforementioned unpleasant symptoms, so be sure to drink plenty of water to minimize discomfort. Just like multivitamins, fiber supplements complement an already balanced diet.

Protein

This is the good one, right? Can't get enough, right? Not so fast. If you eat animal products daily, you probably already consume an adequate amount of protein. If you abstain from eating animal products and do not adequately make up those calories with plant-based protein, you might need to make some changes. If you do eat animal products, then the goal is to keep your proteins lean and incorporate some plant-based proteins to improve the overall quality of your diet.

Animal protein

Chicken
Beef
Pork
Fish
Eggs
Milk/cheese

Plant protein

Beans/Legumes
Soy
Nuts
Peas
Seeds
Whole grains

Nut milk is becoming more popular as an alternative to dairy or soy milk. It is important to note that nut milk is not an adequate source of protein compared to soy or dairy milk. Consider this when substituting nut milk for dairy or soy milk.

Keep animal-based proteins lean by choosing lean cuts of red meat or pork. Remove the skin from chicken before preparation. You may choose to keep the skin on during cooking if you want to enhance flavor with some of the fat from the skin, remove it before eating.

Cooking methods can also affect the fat content of meats. Frying or adding heavy creams or sauces can turn a lean chicken breast into a high-fat entree.

I classify vegetarian or vegan diets into two categories: those that include sufficient plant-based protein and those that don't. We all know someone that does not eat meat, but lentils or chickpeas are nowhere in their pantry.

Fat

Dietary fats are the most nutrient-dense macronutrient at nine calories per gram. There are saturated and unsaturated fats. Saturated fats are in animal products. These are the fats we need to limit in our diet. Avocados are very hot at the moment and a great source of monounsaturated fats. Omega-3 fatty acids found in walnuts, fish, and flaxseed are sources of unsaturated fats. Remember, fats are higher in calories compared to carbohydrates and proteins, so the quantity consumed should be around 20% of total calories (for an 1800 calorie diet, that is 40g of fat daily). Portion sizes are especially important here. It is very easy to consume hundreds of calories of nuts with just a few handfuls.

Water

Drink more water.

Seriously, there is not much to say that you don't already know about proper hydration. The challenge is how that fits into your workday. Consider the following suggestions when seeking to improve your water intake during the day.

Drink a glass of water first thing in the morning, before coffee or any other beverage.

Take a stainless -steel, insulated water bottle with you when you leave the house. Whether you are going to work or going to run errands, you will always have nice, cold water with you. Take a sip when sitting at a traffic light.

Refill your water bottle when you start and finish your breaks at work.

Ask for a water cooler on your unit if it is inconvenient to refill your water bottle between breaks.

Drink water with meals and snacks. Sparkling water is classy and refreshing.

Fresh fruits and vegetables have high water content. Eat them.

Reading nutrition labels

The following are important facts to consider when reading nutrition labels.

"No artificial colors, flavors, or sweeteners."

It sounds good. Surely, we don't want artificial ingredients in our food. However, cane sugar, honey, brown rice or tapioca syrup, salt, and fruit purees are natural ingredients used in place of those artificial ingredients.

These natural ingredients are fine, but when used in excess, they add as many calories and sodium as the fake stuff.

Well RN tip: Don't assume that "no artificial colors, flavors or sweeteners" automatically equals a healthier product.

"No added sugars."

You usually see this on a fruit product. Juice, puree, smoothie or fruit cups. This where a serving size is essential. The nutrition facts panel usually has the serving size listed, and the natural sugar content is per serving. An 8-ounce serving of juice has 28g of sugar. That's seven teaspoons of natural sugars!

Well RN tip: Consume natural fruit sugar in moderation. It's always better to eat the whole fruit because you get more nutritional value, like fiber. If you wish to drink juice, keep it to about 4-6 ounces daily.

"Low sodium" "Reduced sodium" or Lower sodium."

Gold star for you for looking for lower sodium products! The next step is to read the ingredient list and look for sodium replacement: monosodium glutamate or MSG. Yes, the stuff often found in Chinese takeout. You will also find this in processed snacks, frozen foods, or seasoning blends. By the way, 140 mg or less per serving is considered a low sodium product.

Well RN tip: Check the ingredient list for 'monosodium glutamate.' If you find it, don't buy it!

"Low-fat" or Non-fat"

Have you ever thought about how food manufacturers reduce the naturally occurring fat from a food product but still preserve the taste and mouthfeel? Think about products like low-fat or non-fat sour cream, ice creams, yogurts, and protein shakes.

They accomplish this by using food additives called gums like carrageenan, guar, or acacia. When you remove a naturally occurring substance from food, the taste will usually change. Food manufacturers replace it with something to mimic it or mask its absence, like sugar and salt. Fat is the most calorie-dense nutrient, with nine calories per gram and carbohydrates and fat have four calories per gram. Salt has none. When fat is replaced with sugar and salt, mathematically, you will have a lower calorie product.

Well RN tip: When fat is reduced, sugar and salt are likely to be higher in addition to other additives.

"Gluten-Free"

Food marketers rely on your lack of knowledge about gluten. Gluten is in products made from or with wheat, barley, rye, and some oats. There are two kinds of people who care about this label. People with a wheat allergy or have a medically diagnosed intolerance to the wheat proteins that exacerbate Celiac disease, and those who are under the assumption that gluten-free = healthy. Gluten-free products are made with rice, corn, or potato flours and starches. Some oats are gluten-free. Gluten-free products cost more, and some have more sugar and salt added to them than compared to the conventional recipe, which does not make them healthier.

Well RN tip: If you do not have a true allergy or intolerance to wheat, there is no nutritional benefit by avoiding it.

Part 3

Physical activity

What about exercise? Your activity tracker says you burned 400 calories. You use this data as permission to eat a little more than you usually would. Why haven't you lost weight? First, activity trackers are somewhat inaccurate when it comes to estimated calories burned, so take this data lightly. We often underestimate the number of calories we are consuming and overestimating our level of physical activity. Unfortunately, being on your feet and pushing your workstation on wheels up and down the floor for the better part of 8-12 hours does not burn enough calories to gorge on pizza after your shift.

Having a pre-planned physical activity routine is essential to consistency. Try out different activities, days, and times that work well with your work and family schedule. It makes no sense to join a gym when your work hours or family commitments make it nearly impossible to stay consistent. If you don't currently exercise consistently, it will take some adjustment to make room in your schedule for exercise. If you prefer a solo activity, you may need to ask for help from family or friends to make that time for yourself.

You may be asking yourself what counts as physical activity. You don't have to sign up for a marathon, but you do need to challenge your body. That is the ONLY way it will change. Some activities are suitable to get us off our butts and moving, like walking or dancing. However, even those activities can be challenging if performed with the intent to change your body. Home exercise equipment is relatively inexpensive (dumbells, jump rope, mats, weighted exercise balls). There are a plethora of free apps or websites that you can access workout routines to do at home. YouTube is a great place to start. You can create a playlist of short workouts to do right in your living room. Instagram and YouTube are goldmines for bodyweight exercise routines. No gym, no equipment, no problem. I've done quick workouts like these in a hotel room.

Depending on what your budget will allow, you may consider investing in your health by joining a gym or exercise studio. I prefer exercise studios that offer classes that you pay for ahead of time and that do not roll over from month to month. These types of studios tend to be more of an investment than your typical open gyms. Paying a premium has a way of keeping some of us more accountable. No one wants to see their account debited for exercise classes that they don't even use.

According to the 2008 Physical Activity Guidelines for Americans, adults age 18-64 should engage in at least 150 minutes of moderate-intensity aerobic physical activity, 75 minutes of vigorous-intensity aerobic exercise, or a combination of both each week. For substantial weight loss, the time spent doing these activities should double to at least 300 minutes of moderate-intensity physical activity or 150 minutes of vigorous-intensity physical activity per week.

Examples of moderate-intensity activities include gardening, walking 3 miles per hour, playing doubles tennis, or riding a bicycle. Examples of vigorous-intensity activities include jogging, playing singles tennis, hiking up-hill, or jumping rope.

Muscle-strengthening or anaerobic activities are just as crucial as an aerobic activity. Time spent doing muscle-strengthening activities does not count towards time spent doing aerobic exercise. Muscle-strengthening or resistance training is essential to avoiding injury, especially a work-related injury. Without proper core strength, you are more susceptible to a back injury that could keep you from working.

Time, or lack of it, is frequently cited as a barrier to why a person does not exercise. There is no way around having to make time to exercise and putting in the effort to see real change in our bodies. You cannot expect to lose 50 pounds in 6 months if the maximum commitment you are willing to put in is walking around your neighborhood for 30 minutes 3 times a week. This is an excellent start from nothing, but you have to challenge your body if you want it to change. Change is not easy, but once you start seeing results, the sacrifice becomes easier to make. Initially, you may see some weight loss from a moderate increase in physical activity, but your body has a way of adapting and continually needs to be challenged. One day you may do a brisk walk; another day, you may focus on weight training to tone your muscles. Core strength is essential for everyone to prevent lower back injuries. HIIT (high-intensity interval training) is the best way to burn fat in the shortest amount of time. In as little as 20 minutes, you can get in a solid workout provided you put in the maximum effort.

You may have heard of frequency, intensity, time, and type regarding exercise. Modifying one of these elements every time you take time to work out is the key to ensuring variability.

Here is an example of one activity modified three different ways:

Frequency: Walking 30 minutes (2.5-4 miles per hour),

Intensity: 30-second run, 1-minute walk interval for 3o minutes

Time: Walking 50 minutes (2.5-4 miles per hour)

Type: Walking on an incline (3.5-5 incline) for 30 minutes

Monday Walk 30 minutes, 2.5-4 mph

Tuesday 30-second run, 1- minute walk interval for 30 min

Wednesday Rest/Stretch

Thursday Walk at incline 3.5-5 for 30 minutes (challenge: speed intervals)

Friday Rest/Stretch

Saturday 30-second run, 1- minute walk interval for 30 min

Sunday Walk 30 minutes, 2.5-4 mph

Preventing weight gain

Take in fewer calories than you expend. Easier said than done, right? We all know that it is more complicated than that. Several factors affect our ability to prevent weight gain or slow weight loss. Age, stress, medications, and sleep quality are a few. We need to be patient with ourselves when we are starting to make lifestyle changes for weight management. Believe it or not, weight maintenance can be just as hard or harder than weight loss. I often have discussions with clients and patients about the discrepancy between their perceived level of physical activity and their frustrations with a lack of progress. Weight maintenance requires you to maintain a certain level of activity and a sensible diet to prevent weight gain. Weekly weigh-ins are useful to make sure you are staying on track. Of course, slight variations in weight will occur, but if you weigh yourself the same time each week, with the same scale and same clothing (if any), you should be able to see a trend. If your weight starts to trend up without any changes to your lifestyle, then a re-assessment is needed. Weight fluctuations can be related to metabolic changes, medications, or maybe even stress. It would be prudent to follow up with your physician for any unintended weight gain or weight loss to rule out any underlying medical conditions. Some of us would gladly accept unintentional weight loss, but as a nurse, you know this can also be a red flag in health status.

Part 4

Assess your current diet

If you bite it, write it.

Now it's time to reflect on your eating habits to identify the areas that need some work. Record at least three days of whatever you eat. Preferably two workdays and one day off. Include:

- time of day
- where you were eating
- whom you were eating with

You should see patterns in your diet if you are recording honestly.

Analyze your food journal. Where are opportunities for improvement? Are you eating at least three servings of vegetables? How much water are you drinking? What about fruit? At least two servings?

Eating healthier is not just about eating less of something. Sometimes we need to replace the less healthy food with more nutritious choices.

Meal Planning

We all know that our food intake can vary from day to day. Especially on a non-work day to workdays. That is why dietitians ask for a 3-day food diary to account for those variances in food intake. When meal planning, you might want to consider changes in your schedule so you won't be displaced when your schedule changes from one day to the next. You can create a generic meal plan for workdays and non-work days and customize it from week to week.

"A balanced diet is maximizing your nutrient-dense food intake while minimizing food lacking nutritional value." Caryn L. Haywood

Select meals and snacks based on the desired nutrition profile and timing of meals

A lot of nurses have told me they don't know what to eat at work, particularly night shift nurses. I heard a sports nutrition professor say, "eat for what you are going to do, not what you have done." For example, it may be tempting to have a large meal after you have finished a hard workout. However, if you are going to bed a few hours after your workout, you don't need a large meal. Maybe you just got off a 3-11 pm shift and want to eat and go to bed or skip the food altogether. This meal should focus on lean protein and non-starchy vegetables. The same is true if you are getting off the 7 pm to 7 am shift. If you are going to bed, you don't need a high fat or carbohydrate-heavy meal. As tired as you may be, a heavy meal may make it hard for you to fall or stay asleep because the body is busy metabolizing the fat and starch from the meal.

On your way to work? Your pre-work meal may look a little different.

7:00 am
A "normal" breakfast time, but you may find yourself rushing out the door in the morning to clock in on time. Maybe you aren't a "breakfast person" and don't feel like eating in the morning. Two hours into your shift, you are starving and trying to get down to the cafeteria before breakfast service stops. Focus on fruit, lean protein or low-fat dairy and whole grains.

Here are some breakfast ideas:

- Plain Greek yogurt, Ezekiel bread or whole-wheat toast, fruit
- Boiled egg, Ezekiel bread or whole-wheat toast, fruit
- Fruit smoothie made with plain soy milk or Greek Plain yogurt, fruit and oatmeal
- Eggs, oatmeal, and fruit

3 pm or 7 pm shift: This depends on your eating schedule. Your meal right before work should be composed similar to breakfast but with some vegetables. Focus on fruit, lean protein, whole grain or starchy vegetable, and non-starchy vegetables.

Here are some ideas:

- Turkey sandwich on whole wheat bread (lettuce and tomato), carrot sticks, fruit
- Brown rice and beans, salad, fruit
- Chicken or fish, baked potato, fruit

Of course, you have more control when you prepare your meals. However, this requires planning, which some find it challenging to find time to do. What about when you have to choose from the hospital cafeteria? The same rules apply. Water is always the best choice for a beverage. If you drink a caffeinated beverage like coffee, be sure to alternate with water to stay hydrated.

Work snacks!

Proteins and fruit are at the top of my list for snacks. I love trying out new snacks. It's hard for me to walk past snacks in the grocery or drugstore without looking for something new to try.

Let's talk about protein bars. Here is what you want in a protein bar:

Protein: This may sound obvious, but not all protein bars are made equal. Some bars are meal replacements. For snacking purposes, I suggest a protein bar should have at least 7 grams of protein to call itself a protein bar. Any less than that, it's just a snack bar and should be 150 calories or less. If the bar is in the 300-calorie range, it's more of a meal replacement.

Sugar: You want the least amount of *added* sugar as possible, which is different than total carbohydrates. If the bar has fruit in it, it is going to have some natural sugar. You want to minimize the added sugar. A lot of bars advertise low sugar content, but sugar alcohols provide sweetness. Sugar alcohols (xylitol, mannitol, sorbitol) are in sugar-free candies like gum and mints. They have 2.4 calories per gram. They may also cause gastrointestinal distress if consumed in large quantities.

Fiber: This is another nutrient that can vary from bar to bar. Some bars are naturally high in fiber because of the main ingredients, particularly a vegan bar. Other bars may have added fiber like inulin and chicory root. Fiber makes you feel full and helps move waste through your digestive tract. However, too much too soon can make you uncomfortable. Insoluble fiber does not absorb water. Soluble fiber from apples, oats, and flaxseed assist with digestion.

Fat: If your protein bar has nuts, it is going to have high-fat content (more than 5 grams per serving). This is okay. Remember, fat adds twice as many calories per gram than carbohydrates and protein, so nut-based protein bars are naturally going to be higher in calories than a bar without nuts.

Enjoying food for pleasure and stress- eating

Let talk about eating for pleasure. It is okay, in moderation. Being a wine and chocolate lover myself, I am all about enjoying food and drink strictly for fun. For a lot of people, holidays are a pain point when it comes to trying to eat healthily. Hence, the common new year's resolution to eat healthier and lose weight. Allow yourself to enjoy food, within reason. It's okay to have a few bites of cake instead of a whole slice. I always feel super proud of myself when I can throw away a piece of candy or bag of chips without finishing it. It means I have control over my cravings. Emotional eating will get us into trouble if it is not acknowledged and addressed. I am not immune to emotional eating. It's essential to plan for those times that you know you will be vulnerable to eating out of stress. It's okay to snack, for the right reasons, and with better choices. Yes, I know there will be days when only a Snickers bar will do. Just be sure that these days are exceptions and not the standard snack choice. You can probably identify times during your typical work shift where you find yourself searching for a snack and end up in front of a vending machine or looking for leftover sweets in the hospital conference room.

Part 5

Weight loss

Its mind-blowing how much money is spent every year on weight-loss programs, supplements, procedures, exercise programs, and more. According to fooducate.com, 75 million Americans are actively trying to lose weight, and the average person spends about $800 a year trying to do so. All with the target outcome of weight loss. Desirable weight is a pain point for many. It is crucial to be realistic with our expectations for a goal weight. Sometimes weight may not be the issue but rather body composition. I'm sure that you have heard that weight loss takes time. You did not gain 20 pounds overnight, so don't expect to lose 20 pounds overnight. You can only restrict calories so much, especially if you are a working adult. You need your energy to perform daily tasks without succumbing to hypoglycemia! Physical activity is so important. It allows you to burn those calories needed to create a significant enough deficit for weight loss. A sustainable physical activity regimen is necessary to maintain consistency for weight reduction. What is a sustainable physical activity regimen for you? Everyone will be different. Maybe you co-parent and use the time that your children are not home to focus on your self-care. Perhaps you have a partner that supports your efforts by stepping up to watch the children so you can take an hour for yourself 3-4 times a week. You may go outside the home for exercise or slip into a spare room without any interruptions. You may need to communicate with your partner or other family members that you need their help to create some self-care time, and you can reciprocate for them as well.

As mentioned earlier, we tend to overestimate our level of physical activity, especially if you have an activity tracker that you use for motivation. These energy expenditure calculators are not as accurate as we would like them to be, but they do serve as good reminders for us to get up and move!
Create a physical activity routine. Keep in mind your current commitments. However, you must make this a priority. How do you currently spend your time? Take time to reflect on a typical workday and a typical day off.

Weight can be tricky when it comes down to a single number. Sometimes we can get fixated on a certain weight. If a patient or client tells me they want to lose weight, and they have a particular weight in mind, I will ask them a few questions regarding that weight. First, when was the last time they were at that weight, if ever. Second, I will ask about other "numbers" that will demonstrate improvement in health status. Numbers like cholesterol, blood pressure, blood sugar, and even waist circumference can also give a measurable number to monitor health status beyond weight. For reference, here are some numbers beyond your weight that you should know to monitor your health status.

Cholesterol: <200 mg/dL

Triglycerides: <150 mg/dL

Fasting blood sugar: 65-99 mg/dL

Blood pressure: systolic **less** than 120 and diastolic **less** than 80 mmHg

Healthy and obese?

There has been much conversation regarding the topic of health versus body size. Recently, a critic wrote an article bashing Nike's plus-sized mannequin, suggesting obesity and fitness cannot exist in the same body. Some believe that promoting this minimizes obesity's overall impact on health. Proponents of body acceptance believe that someone can be clinically overweight or obese, but otherwise healthy. I implore you to engage in an honest reflection about your body image and how you feel about your body size and health status. As a nurse, you may have to bring up the issue with your patients. The more comfortable you are with your self-image, the more supportive and objective you can be when having that conversation.

Mental Health

"Comparison is the thief of joy."

I am so happy that mental health is being discussed more in mainstream media these days. The connection between our physical health and mental health is undeniable. I believe that anyone who has provided patient care in any setting has witnessed the contrast of a person with a positive mental attitude and someone emanating negative energy and the impact on their health status. Think of a cancer patient who is optimistic about their treatment and recovery versus a person whose ailments are a direct result of poor lifestyle choices due to a lack of self-love and efficacy.

Nutrition plays a significant role in our mental health. If we are feeling good about ourselves and are functioning from a place of self-love, we will nourish our body with healthy food. Sometimes we "treat" ourselves to foods that are high in saturated fat and sugar because we have had a hard day, and the consumption of these food triggers a self-soothing emotion that feels like self-care. It is essential to recognize this dangerous habit. If we get conditioned to reward ourselves with food, even nourishing food, it may lead to a mismanaged relationship with food.

Social Media

You might be asking yourself why I put these two together. Social media has taken over almost every aspect of our lives. Most people have at least one social media profile, even if it is just a LinkedIn account. We use social media to keep in touch with friends and family that we are too busy to see as much we like. Some of us want to use social media apps for lifestyle motivation and inspiration. I am thankful that I remember a time when we didn't have a camera in our hands at every moment.
I mentioned earlier that a digital vision board via Pinterest might help you visualize how you want your life to look. However, we must be careful not to fall into the comparison trap when it comes to social media. It is easy to stumble upon a social media account and start comparing yourself to someone who you have never met based on carefully curated and staged photos on their Instagram or Facebook page.

When trying to make positive lifestyle changes, I believe it is good to have a sound support system, but be careful not to compare yourself to others. Especially on social media. Everyone puts their best foot forward on social media. If you have ever posted a picture of yourself on social media, you probably took several hundred photos to find the one worthy of posting, right? Okay, maybe not

several hundred, but you get the idea. Don't compare your daily challenges to an imagined near-perfect life that you see on social media. You may not even realize that you are comparing yourself to others in this way. Try this, next time you get on social media, check with how you feel about yourself before and after. You might realize that you are more anxious or self-conscious after looking at other people's profiles. If this happens to you, you may need to take a break from social media to gain perspective of your reality. Perfect pictures and reposted quotes are not #goals. Goals are what makes you truly happy, regardless if others share those same goals or even approve of your goals. I liken it to putting on blinders.
Stay focused on you and how you feel about yourself. Don't let social media fool you into thinking that you have to share every detail about your life or that the value of the moments that you share is based on the number of likes or praiseworthy comments you receive. I recently went to an adults-only "summer camp." The best part of the camp was that there was almost no cellular or wifi service, so making calls, texting, and checking social media was not an option for 72 hours. Everyone engaged with each other. Some people had their phones out to take pictures, but for the most part, most people left their phones in the bunks. It was so liberating to be able to fellowship and enjoy nature without technology diluting the experience.

If sharing your weight loss journey or healthy meal choices motivates you to keep up with lifestyle changes, by all means, share.

Identifying Unique Challenges and Eliminating Excuses

You may be thinking to yourself that you understand that exercise and proper diet are both critical components to achieving or maintaining a healthy weight. But what does all this mean to you as a nurse? Your schedule changes from day-to-day, and you might plan your work schedule around a family members' calendar.

Take a step back and remember that you are your priority. You cannot pour from an empty cup. Let's not forget the mental and emotional health benefits of taking care of our bodies. Have you ever regretted a workout? No? Why? Because even though you may not have wanted to start in the first place, you cannot deny the fact that your mood improved from a workout. Exercise produces 'feel good' hormones. Imagine how your mood and energy levels would be different if you were consistent and intentional with your workouts.

Think about it; you are going about your day, everything is fine, usual work tasks, nothing too out of the ordinary. Then it happens, a demanding family member of one of your patients starts asking you a bunch of questions that are really out of your scope of practice to answer. The patient has a million consults out; only one specialist has come to see the patient. It's 9 am, you don't have all the answers, and they are taking it out on you. Your lunch break finally rolls around, and you are hoping they are serving those amazing fried chicken wings and fries in the cafeteria because a salad won't feel as good as crispy wings and fries with ketchup and mayo.

Maybe you work the overnight shift. You did not get as much rest as you wanted to because of family drama. You managed to eat at home before you came to work but forgot to bring a snack. It looks like it is going to be break room coffee and vending machine chips and a candy bar for you tonight.

These are two examples of situations that may occur that can thwart the best of intentions to eat healthier. We all have daily triggers that arise that have to potential to knock us off our game. The key is to identify them so that you can plan and lessen the likelihood that you will make less than the best choice for your nutrition.
Think about the last time you set out to make better nutrition or lifestyle choices, and things did not go as planned. Can you pinpoint what the trigger was that made things go left? Is there a situation that you frequently encounter that you find yourself always reacting to instead of being proactive?
Now think about how you can be proactive and set yourself up to win the next time you encounter

these challenging situations or triggers. How will you hold yourself accountable for making the healthier choice? Will you report to a friend or co-worker what you ate for lunch or snack that day? Will you journal it on paper or using an app on your phone? We will discuss this in more detail later on, but for now, think about how you can set yourself up to win!

Support system

Who is your support system?
Is it a friend or relative? A fellow nurse? Group chats? Facebook? Will you be creating a picture diary on Instagram? It would be wise to have two sources of support, so you do not always depend on one method. Decide how often you will check-in and share it with your support partner or partners. If you decide to document your progress digitally, feel free to use the hashtag #wellRN.

Creating lasting lifestyle changes

Action Plan

- Identify what you want to improve. Be as specific as possible. You want your success to be measurable.

- Identify current barriers.

- Identify ways to overcome these barriers.

- Create a system for success. What actions **must** you take to make achieving your goal as effortless as possible? The easier it is to succeed, the easier it will be to maintain.

- How much time are you going to give yourself to meet your goal? It helps to plan for re-assessment at least once. Sometimes methods we think are great do not turn out to be as practical as we thought they would be.

Conclusion

It is vital to know that we are all a work in progress. You will start, stop, start over, stop, and pick up where you left off. Hopefully, each time you start over, you remember what did not work the previous times and start something different. We are striving to be the best version of ourselves and allowing mistakes and learning opportunities are a part of the process. Trust that with intentional care for your well-being; you can look in the mirror and say to yourself, "I am a Well RN."

Made in the USA
Monee, IL
05 November 2026

67962923R00031